What Not To Do in Beauty for the Mature Woman

Rose Rubio

NEWMAN SPRINGS PUBLISHING
320 Broad Street
Red Bank, NJ 07701

First originally published by
Newman Springs Publishing 2023

ISBN 979-8-88763-110-3 (Paperback)
ISBN 979-8-88763-111-0 (Digital)

Printed in the United States of America

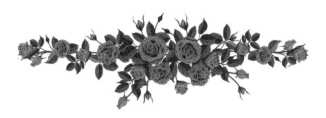

ACKNOWLEDGMENT

I would like to thank my dear friend Blair for sending me a text two years ago, telling me, "Rose, you need to put all that knowledge you have in a book!" At the time, I just laughed, but one and a half years later, I started writing 😊.

Thank you, Blair, for always believing in me!

I was cutting my friend Lisa's hair and telling her of my writing this book. I then told her I was looking for a proofreader. She turned around and said to me, "Rose, I can do that for you! I do it all the time where I work!"

Thank you, Lisa, for your talent and time spent doing this for me 😊. *You are a godsent angel!*

After writing this book, I needed an editor. I spoke to several editors and did not jive with any of them. I prayed for the good Lord to help me find the right person. Two weeks after my last attempt to find an editor, a former client from twenty years ago, Toni Taylor Glenn, came into the salon for a haircut. We had lost touch after I had moved to Boston. A mutual friend had told her I was back.

Toni had edited my first book, *A Touch Tells All*. When I saw her, I knew my prayers had been answered. She already knew me, my work, and my passion for fashion and beauty. My prayers were answered.

Thank you, Toni, for putting this information together in a way that all women can understand. You are a beautiful soul and a wonderful writer. I appreciate all the time and energy you put into this. I could not have completed this without you!

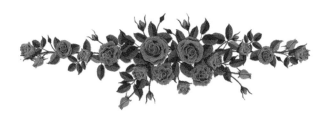

INTRODUCTION

As the door to my salon played its welcoming chime, a new client in her mid-fifties walked in and looked around the room. I greeted her and invited her to take a seat, while I finished up with the woman still in my chair.

I couldn't help but notice that her look was *all wrong* for her. This is what I am trained to do as a beauty coach, fashion designer, and hairstylist.

Actually, she looked just like the many mature women I see every day, trying to wear the latest trends. Unfortunately, many wear them in ways that are not flattering to them. There is no one size or one look that fits all.

Trends have always been with us in every aspect of the beauty business. Whether it's the latest in skin care, hair, makeup, or fashion, trends come and go and then come back again slightly different.

I've also learned that most women look to the media to tell them what colors to wear and how to apply the latest trend in lipstick or eye makeup, regardless of their own canvas. Your canvas is the composite of your skin tone and texture, hair type and color, face shape, body shape, features, and personality. Everyone's canvas is uniquely theirs.

Media only cares about selling the products, not about how to teach people to incorporate them into their own personal style.

So come with me as we take a look at some simple ways to adapt the latest trends in hair, fashion, and makeup. And more importantly, *what not to do*, when putting together *your* best look.

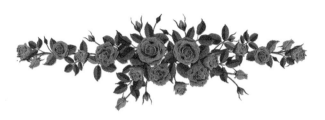

IS YOUR IMAGE
A REFLECTION OF
WHO YOU ARE?

When considering a new hairstyle or fashion trend, it's important to remember that your image or style should be intentional! It's your signature. With so many products and choices, you can create whatever look that fits for you—from warm and inviting to funky, natural, or more conservative.

Start with your best you! Beautiful hair and skin are your foundation and the direct result of a healthy body and lifestyle. They take nourishment from the food, vitamins, minerals, and moisture that you take into your body. The following are healthy habits everyone should practice to have lustrous hair and healthy glowing skin:

- Eat a healthy, balanced diet, and drink plenty of water for hydration.
- Limit sugar, alcohol, and caffeine intake to moderate levels.
- Get enough rest and sleep to avoid puffiness and dark circles around your eyes.

When your skin is not healthy and hydrated, no amount of makeup can conceal it or make it look better.

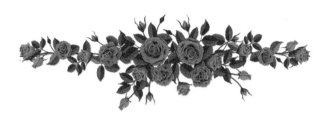

CHAPTER 1

A Closer Look at Skin Care

When we're young, we take our smooth, flawless skin for granted. But as we age, we need a good skin care regimen. It can be very simple: cleanse, moisturize, and tone, preferably with natural ingredients, rather than chemicals.

If you wish to add a serum to your regimen, you can. I use jojoba oil (lightweight) under my eyes. You can also use a night cream or glycolic acid to achieve a brighter, smoother, clearer-looking skin.

I personally like to use a microcurrent device that will circulate the blood and oxygen and collagen to the surface of my skin. With a microcurrent device, you are constantly nurturing your skin. I use mine three times a week, ten to fifteen minutes each time. It is amazing how it diminishes lines and keeps your skin plump and feeling soft naturally. Also, use sunscreen, and do not use too much spray tan.

Foundation

When applying makeup, use a foundation closest to your skin tone. The most important tip I can give you is that *less is more*! Too much makeup is unattractive and emphasizes your lines.

Always use an upward movement, and use less as you get to your hairline, ears, and neck. Blend in thoroughly so your skin will look smooth. Whether you use a brush, sponge, or finger-tips, use a light touch and outward movement.

If your skin is dry, use a moisturizer as a primer under your foundation. If you do not want a heavy thick finish, try using a tinted moisturizer, or add drops of water to your foundation for light coverage.

Eye Makeup

When using eye makeup, always remember light colors bring out your features and make them look more pronounced. Dark colors make them less pronounced.

As we age, we should stay away from shiny shadows and powders. You can still do some trendy-looking eyes, but use matte finish products.

To achieve brighter eyes, stick with matte, nude shades around the eyes, and use a very light (ivory or

nude) liner on your lower lid, some-
times referred to as our waterline.

Neutral colors are the best for a
youthful look. When using eye shadows, don't use your own eye color.
Example: Do not use blue eyeshadow
on blue eyes. Try using the opposite
color on the color board to compliment your eye color. Keep in mind…
less is always more.

Eyelashes/Eyeliner

If you wear false eyelashes, you
want them to be natural looking and
cut to fit your eyes. Any makeup artist
can show you how to cut them to the

right size. Also, use a dark-tone eyelash glue to achieve an illusion of eyeliner.

As we get older, using less liner is a good thing. Using eyeliner to completely outline your eyes will make them look smaller. Simply brush an uplifting line in the corner of your eye with brow shadow. You can also place three dots of liner along the lower lid and smudge them.

Here's a story to demonstrate my point:

One day a good friend showed up for her appointment—straight from having her makeup done in a department store by someone from a prominent makeup line from New York. I looked at her and gasped, "OMG! What have you done to your face?"

She had shiny, sparkling blue eyeshadow from her eyelids to her eyebrows! I could not see her pretty blue eyes. All I could see was the shadow. It was not a good look!

As she came closer, I could see a very thick foundation, caked with lots of shiny powder, which emphasized her lines when she smiled. And the blush was too dark for her fair skin. I knew whoever did this to her was just trying to sell her a lot of products.

After explaining why this was not a good look for her, I suggested she return the makeup and get a refund.

Lessons to be learned: Stay with your natural skin color. Use complimentary colors on your eyes, and less is more.

Eyebrows

Eyebrows are very important to open up your eyes. Be sure to have them shaped to your face, and be careful not to get them too thin or too thick. If you want your eyes to look bigger, your brow must be well shaped and not too thick toward the center of your face.

Also, keep the color of your eyebrows as close as you can to your natural hair color.

If you use a gel to fill in your eyebrow, use it sparingly. A great filler is eyeshadow. I use dark brown. My natural hair color is dark brown.

Microbladed eyebrows are another way to achieve natural-looking brows. The difference is they will not wash away at night when you wash your face.

Here's an eyebrow nightmare!

When a friend of mine was in her teens, she told me that she turned to teen magazines to tell her how to look glamorous. A cover photo of one of her favorite movie stars revealed thin, arched eyebrows. *That's what I want to look like*, she thought! She got the tweezers and went to work on her thick, wide eyebrows.

The next day at school, her friends tried to conceal their laughter as they asked, "What have you done to your eyebrows?" Her new look was all wrong for her face and the shape of her eyes. Her copycat strategy had failed, and she was miserable, waiting for them to grow back out.

> *Lesson learned: Stay with your
> natural shape and canvas.*

Lipstick

When applying lipstick, use a lip liner to outline the shape of your lips. Always use a liner color close to your lipstick. The lip liner will keep your lipstick from smudging over your lip line.

If you have a lot of lines around your lips, it is very important to stay away from dark colors, which bring attention to this area.

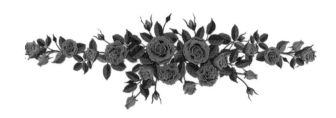

CHAPTER 2

Focusing on Hair

As I have stressed, real beauty begins from within. No hairstyle or color can conceal unhealthy, dry, or lifeless hair. Over the years, I have developed the ability to diagnose illness, imbalances, or changes in our bodies that affect the strength and texture of hair close to the scalp. This was the subject of my first book, *Touch Tells All*.

Here's an example.

A long-time client came in for a perm. After getting shampooed, I felt the hair next to her scalp and immediately knew something had changed: it was very depleted and lifeless. When I told her I could not put chemicals on depleted hair, she said that I had to be wrong. She said she had just been to her doctor, and all her tests came back good.

"Then you have to be pregnant," I said, which she quickly denied. I still refused the perm, which did not make her happy. However, a little over a month later, she returned and announced that she was six weeks pregnant—with twins! From the very beginning of her pregnancy, the fetuses had been absorbing all her nutrients, causing the depletion in her hair.

Medications, alcohol, stress, surgery or serious illness, and poor diet will also deplete the hair.

Hair must be strong and healthy to be able to respond to chemicals such as color and perms. Otherwise, chemicals leave it frayed, more weakened, and dull. Healthy hair will also have more body, shine, and strength.

When making positive or happy lifestyle changes, the increased oxygen, hormones, and circulation can make a positive difference in hair health too. It all shows up in the first inch of your hair. I can tell when my single clients are delighting in a new relationship!

Lesson to be learned: Hair tells all!

Whether your hair is short, medium length, or long, always try to have soft, flowing movement. This means no heavy hairspray that makes it stiff. Helmet hair will age you more than anything. The natural movement of your hair will give you the illusion of youth.

The hard reality is that as we age, we develop lines on our forehead, bags under eyes, creases from nose to chin, and lines around our mouth. But here's the good news: simply styling your hair upward and back from your face will de-emphasize your lines and give an uplifting illusion.

You can also use soft bangs if you have a high forehead.

Here are examples of what not to do in styling hair:

- Do not wear your hair down and around your face.
- Stay away from flat straight hair because it brings the illusion of all movement down.
- If you have a long neck, don't style your hair going toward the center of your neck. Keep it at shoulder length with back-

ward movement. Otherwise, it will draw attention to the lines on your neck.

- Do not part the hair in the middle if you have a prominent or crooked nose. The part brings direct attention to the nose.
- Do not part your hair on the side if you have a square face.

Just remember not to do anything that may emphasize or bring attention to features you may want to minimize, like prominent ears, nose, chin, or aging lines!

Fortunately, women today have lots of options!

Now, here's a can-do list!

Women with a short neck can wear a short bob with lots of elevation for an upward movement, which is created by adding layers. Short hair will also give the illusion of a longer neck. So always keep in mind the results you want.

Women with an average neck can wear many styles.

Go with the natural movement of your hair. Whether you have curly, wavy, or straight hair, it will be a lot easier for you to manage if you go with its natural movement. If you have curly hair, you will also avoid damage from the heated tools used to straighten it.

Gray hair can feel and look youthful, if you wear it short and "spiky."

Shorter hair will look better 85 percent of the time, as long as it is soft and wispy.

Another flattering style for gray hair is to wear it long on top and short in the back. With this style, you can create soft and flowing movement over one eye. Or you can use a strong gel and light hairspray and dry your hair backward to create a deep, chic wave look. Another option to feel unique and chic is to try an asymmetrical cut with volume and movement throughout.

The classic bob looks great on faces with minimal lines. Also, the angled bob with layers and soft bangs is flattering.

There are many other things you can do to minimize or soften features that aren't your favorites, such as the following:

- If you have a prominent or crooked nose, you should off-center the part on the right or left, depending on which direction the tip of your nose goes.
- If the tip of your nose goes to the right, you want to part your hair on the right side and move the hair to the left.
- Also stay away from heavy bangs. Showing your forehead will de-emphasize your nose.

- If you have a round-shaped face, try creating a square shape with the haircut and style.
- If you have a heart-shaped face, wear full bangs with full sides from your cheekbone to chin.
- If your face is rectangular, do not wear your hair straight down. Create a round effect with the haircut and style.
- Oval faces can wear just about any style! Just don't cover up your face with hair. Show that pretty shape!

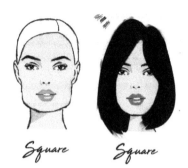

Square   *Square*

SQUARE-SHAPED FACE—
CREATE ROUND ILLUSION WITH HAIR

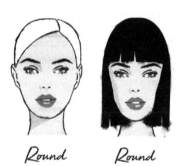

Round   *Round*

ROUND-SHAPED FACE—
CREATE SQUARE ILLUSION WITH HAIR

WHAT NOT TO DO IN BEAUTY FOR THE MATURE WOMAN

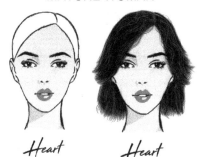

Heart   *Heart*

HEART-SHAPED FACE—CREATE OVAL ILLUSION WITH HAIR

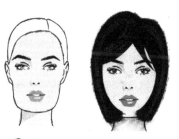

Rectangle   *Rectangle*

RECTANGULAR-SHAPED FACE— CREATE ILLUSION OF OVAL WITH SHORT LAYERED BOB

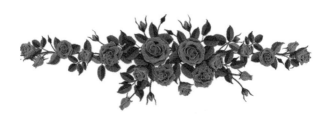

CHAPTER 3

Hair Coloring

Ninety percent of the time, the natural color you were born with will be the best color for your skin tone.

If you decide to change your hair color, try to stay within two shades lighter or darker than your natural color. You can add more warmth or depth but try to stay within two shades of difference.

Going Blonde

If you want to go very light blonde, *expect damage*! Bleach can break down the hair shaft or cuticle to a point of stretching or breaking off! Then your ends look dry, frazzled, and brittle. Always discuss achieving a darker or multiple shades of blonde with your hairdresser.

The lighter you go with the color, the more damage you will have to your hair. Also, going too light will make you look older. Multicolor blondes or soft-color brunettes are a better look for mature women, and they are probably closer to your skin tone.

Here's a story of "Blonde Gone Bad":

The first time I saw this client in Oklahoma City, I felt really bad for her because of what someone had done to her overbleached, permed hair. She looked up at me with her big, beautiful eyes and asked, "So what do you think?"

I smiled at her and said, "I not only say no to this bleached, permed hair—I say *hell no*."

She let out a sigh of relief and a smile.

I told her we could fix this, but
my first goal is to get her hair healthy
again. Second is to cut her hair in a
style that is best for her face shape.
My third goal is to create a color that
would bring out her beautiful skin
tone, because the bleach blonde made
her look washed out.

I immediately did two different
conditioning treatments and gave her
protein and moisture treatments to
use at home. Then I cut her hair to
a more flattering style, and we made
an appointment for two weeks to get
color.

When she returned, we were both
excited to feel the difference in her
hair. I chose a light reddish-brown

for her color and added lowlights, the reverse of highlights. I needed the red to absorb into the previously bleached hair, and reddish brown was a beautiful color for her skin tone.

In three months of continuous treatment, her hair was restored to health and beauty!

That was thirty-five years ago. The fun part of this story is that today, we are still friends, and I still do her hair.

Leave the "trendy colors" to the younger generation. The pink, blue, green, and ashy gray trends cause lots of damage, but when we are young… do we care?

For the most part, women over forty, for whom this book is written, look best in pretty, shiny, healthy, and softer hair.

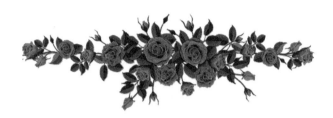

CHAPTER 4

Let's Talk about Products

Shampoo and Conditioner

When your hair gets stripped by shampoos that open the cuticle, you will lose your color and also enhance frizz, if your hair is prone to frizzing. Here's a good test. If your hair feels squeaky clean after a shampoo, it has been

stripped. Make sure to do this test,
or consult your hairdresser before you
apply conditioner.

When using conditioners, look for
one that actually penetrates into the
hair. Most conditioners will just coat
the hair. You can test it by putting a
dime-size amount in the palm of your
hand and rubbing it into your hands,
top and bottom. If it absorbs into the
skin and feels hydrated, it is a good
conditioner! If it looks and feels oily on
your skin, it will not penetrate or moisturize your hair. Oil-based products
will make your hair shiny, but they do
not add moisture.

Oil-based products are not bad. It
just depends on what you are trying to

achieve. If you are looking for shine, oily products will achieve that.

Always keep in mind what your needs are before you purchase products.

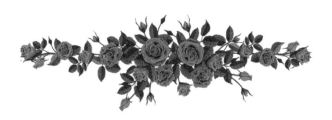

CHAPTER 5

Top it all off with the right fashion for you!

Connecting your self-confidence to your style feels liberating. Heads up, shoulders back—you are ready to take on the world! Or at least the challenge du jour!

Fabrics and Colors

We are blessed with an abundance of lovely fabrics, colors, and textures to choose from when building our wardrobes.

Here are a few suggestions:

- The fabric of your garments should not be stiff! When picking out an outfit, look for fabrics that are soft and flowing, like I suggested with hair (soft and flowing).
- If the fabric is stiff, it will make you appear larger than you really are! If you have an area

you do not wish to emphasize, wear soft, loose fabrics.

- As for colors, stay away from muted colors. Look for bright, bold colors that look good with your skin tone and will give you an uplift.
- If you are uncomfortable with bold colors, try mixing with soft pastels. You can add one bold color to soft pastels, as well as adding a pastel to an outfit with lots of bold colors!
- By mixing and matching colors, you can create what is comfortable and flattering for you. This is how to use trendy

colors and adapt them to fit your canvas.
• Keep in mind, if your waist is smaller than your hips, wearing a belt can give you a nice silhouette.

When It Comes to Styles

Only women with large breasts should wear V-neck sweaters and tops. Women with small breasts can wear round collars or turtlenecks to give them the illusion of larger breasts, if they wish.

If you wear glasses, look for a design that flatters the shape of your face as well as the trend.

Do not wear a belt if you have a large waist.

Do not wear tight clothing unless you are toned. Do not get too busy with patterns and colors. If you wear a jumpsuit that has multicolors, you can wear a solid, preferably dark blazer or a long topcoat that picks up one of the colors. The solid dark tone will give a slenderizing illusion.

Another beautiful look is solid black underneath a red blazer or long topcoat. Then add a scarf with lots of bright colors. You can create the same effect with pastel colors!

When choosing colors to wear, stay away from anything that is close to your skin tone—because this combination will wash you out. For example, people with pale skin should not wear white. Dark-skinned women should not wear brown.

Watch out for floral designs and tweeds, which can be somewhat aging or make you look larger (depending on size of print). In my opinion, floral patterns *never* look sexy regardless of age!

If you want to project a little bit of sexy, always just give a hint rather than overexpose your body!

If you wear panty hose or stockings, try to stay close to your natural skin tone, unless you are wearing black. Black is always sexy!

One rule of thumb to keep from looking frumpy: keep your silhouettes opposite of each other, with tops loose and bottoms tight *or* tops tight and bottoms loose.

"Look Good, Feel Better!"

The above heading is borrowed from the American Cancer Society, which created a program to provide wigs to women who had lost their hair to chemo or radiation. They called it *Look Good, Feel Better*—because it works!

It's important to take an interest in your appearance at any age. When you neglect your appearance, you can limit your potential. It can also lead to or aggravate depression. It's like giving up on yourself, on life, and on all its possibilities.

Taking time to care for yourself and look your best gives you confidence to be open to all of life's opportunities. Once you get your first compliment, you will be amazed how much better you will feel!

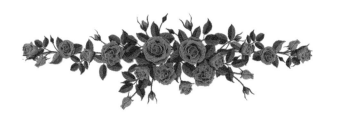

WHAT TO WEAR FOR DIFFERENT SHAPES

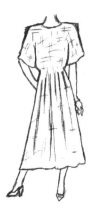

Small Shoulders, Large Hips?

With this body shape, it is good to bring emphasis on the shoulders, whether that be with shoulder pads or pattern design.

You now have created an illusion of a smaller waist and better silhouette of your body.

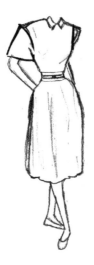

Straight Lines

If you have more straight lines,
you can put an emphasis on shoulders,
as well as wear a belt to give the illusion of curves.

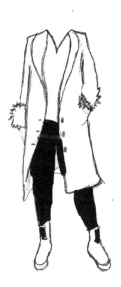

Larger Size from Waist to Hip Area

Bring emphasis on shoulders, and wear straight longer style tops or blazers. Stay away from short jackets.

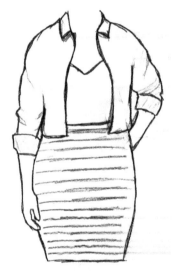

This is an example of what not to do if you have small shoulders and large hips.

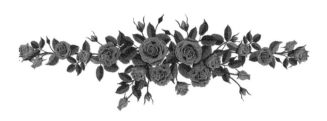

WHAT ABOUT
HANDBAGS?

Here's the rule of thumb for handbags:

Small frame	=	Small bag
Large frame	=	Large bag
M e d i u m frame	=	M e d i u m bag

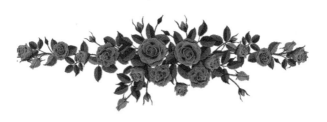

SOME PARTING
THOUGHTS

There is a timeless, universal truth that has been with us since humans began handing down wisdom in both spoken and written words: *Moderation in all things*.

As I have tried to demonstrate, moderation is important in creating the most healthy, flattering look in all aspects of beauty.

We have a constant stream of fun, new trends in the beauty and fashion world! Play with them, embrace them, enjoy them! But remember to always *individualize* to your own unique style—to the canvas that is you!

I hope this book will be helpful to you in creating the image that best reflects your true beauty, your best features, and your style—especially as we age! With this guide, you can always look your best!

And most importantly, always remember to smile because that puts a sparkle in your eyes and a lift in your face and in your step! Your smile is the icing on your beautifully crafted cake!

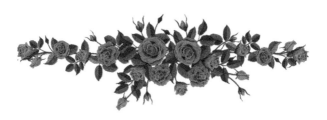

ABOUT THE AUTHOR

Rose Rubio has been a nationally recognized beauty consultant, hairstylist, makeup artist, and fashion designer for more than fifty years. Her passion has been not only staying on top of trends and fashions but also teaching her clients ways to adapt them to always look their best.

Early in her early career in the sixties, Rose trained with legendary fashion and hairstyling icons, like Vidal

Sassoon in San Francisco and Paul Mitchell in New York City. She has earned her place on the leading edge of this fast-changing industry, designing and managing her own award-winning, innovative salons for twenty-five of those years.

One of her salons, *The Place to Be*, was written up in *National Salon Magazine* as the first spá in the Midwest to offer all beauty and fashion services in one place.

Rose's foray into fashion design was inspired by her desire to help a friend, who was a talented performer and wore a size 16. Her friend had a difficult time finding stylish gowns over a size 12. Rose started designing gowns that complimented her friend's best features, minimized her body size, and brought out her personality!

Soon other friends and clients wanted Rose's designs. By popular demand, her work was showcased in her fashion show—*A Touch of Rose*—featuring casual wear, evening wear, and coats. Each guest received a long-stemmed rose, which is still her signature logo today.

Rose has compiled her expertise in this coaching course for mature women. Here, you will discover simple ways to enhance your unique beauty with vibrant hair, glowing skin, and complimentary styles and colors. This is her art, her passion, and her gift to you!

Printed in the USA
CPSIA information can be obtained
at www.ICGtesting.com
LVHW071146090224
771310LV00020B/520